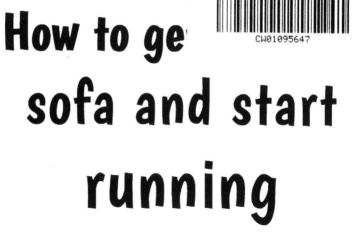

How to get off the sofa and start running

by
Annie Page

Second Edition

Published by and available from
theendlessbookcase.com

The Endless Bookcase Ltd
71 Castle Road, St Albans, Hertfordshire,
England, UK, AL1 5DQ.

Printed Edition
Also available in multiple e-book formats.

ISBN: 978-1-912243-02-0

This one's for Goldie xx

Reviews

"If you are new to running this is a basic beginners guide to getting started. It will cover all your questions about where to start and how to start. The author Annie has written this from her heart, enlightening others from her own experiences as a beginner. Now a regular runner and coach she now hopes to help others embarking on their own running campaign."

Liz Yelling – Double Olympian and Commonwealth Bronze Medalist.

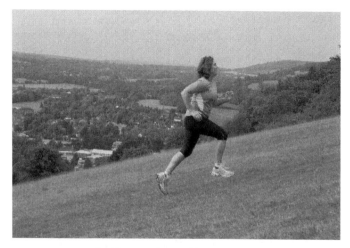

Annie running at Box Hill

'This made me think that even I could run 5k ... A concept never considered before...'
Tes Smith

'Lovely light tone and gets across the important messages.'
Madeleine Tate

'Never having run before I am now feeling inspired and motivated to put the running plan into practice!'
Lucy Hampton

About the Author

Annie Page is a qualified UK Athletics Running Coach, an *NLP* Trainer and Master Practitioner and a Coaching Master – who really enjoys running!

"I had not run since leaving school, where I was probably one of the few who actually enjoyed cross country. I started running again in 2004, with a friend and we started off not being able to run for more than a couple of minutes and then needing to walk, which was great because the plan we were following told us to do just that (there is one at the end of the book).

From there I fell back in love with running...

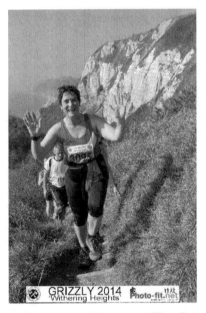

Coming up Stairway to Heaven at The Grizzly 2014

More at the back....

Highlighted Words

There are a few pieces of jargon, technical or scientific terms used in this book and they are highlighted in *italics* (see NLP above) – all these terms are explained at the end of the book.

Those words highlighted in **bold and italics** are references to companies, people, clubs etc.

Contents

Why Run?

"The miracle isn't that I finished. The miracle is that I had the courage to start."

~ John Bingham

People start running for many different reasons, they want to lose weight, get fit, beat stress or, like me, you like eating chocolate.

Running has many benefits and it is one of the best exercises you can do to improve the physical conditioning of your heart and lungs. It is proven as one of the best fat burning exercises and it is estimated that people burn an average of 100 calories per mile run – although this does depend on your weight, your speed, your intensity and the terrain!

There are also very strong links with helping people deal with stress, mild depression and emotional strain. There is growing research which shows that exercise may be as effective as anti-depression medication, in some cases. Exercise releases *endorphins* (the feel good chemical) from the brain. **The Mayo Clinic** puts exercise at the top of its list of ways to relieve stress

Running is convenient and low on equipment needed making it accessible to almost everyone, especially those just starting out. Although that's not to say that as you get more into your running you can't buy many and varied items to help with your training, racing, wardrobe and shoe collection! (I know many men who have far more shoes than me if you include their running shoes...)

Running can be as social or as solitary as you want it to be, both have great benefits. I love running with my club mates for the company, to catch up with everyone, maybe to push me a bit further, or being with them as they reach their own goals. I also love the time I get to spend on my own, around the beautiful countryside that we have, using the time to think through what I need to do for work, planning my day or just letting my mind have some time off.

Whatever your reasons for starting running the rewards you get from it will be powerful and long lasting both physically and mentally.

Happy Running!

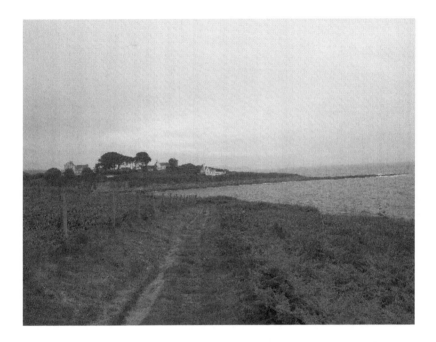

South West Coastal Path, Cornwall

The basic equipment you will need

"I decided to go for a little run."

~ Forrest Gump

When you start out running you do not need to worry about lots of expensive equipment. The basics you need are a proper pair of running shoes and for the ladies a good sports bra. As you progress you may want to invest in some running specific clothing.

Shoes

These will be your first consideration and your biggest commitment in money terms, so it is important to get it right. There are many different types of running shoes and you want a pair that works for your running style, so you need to go to a specialist running shop rather than on line – there are now quite a lot around the country from independents to nationwide. At a specialist shop the staff can advise you and will watch you run in different shoes, either on a treadmill or in the shop. You may feel slightly silly or daft if you've not done this before but by doing this they can make sure you get the right shoes and the right fit – not necessarily the most expensive ones!

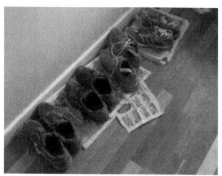

When you are buying your running shoes you may find that they are a bigger size than what you would normally wear. This is because your feet will swell slightly when running and so it can be better to buy shoes in the afternoon as your feet will be slightly bigger and closer to how they will feel on a run.

Sports Bra

It can not only be very uncomfortable to have too much movement when running, but it can also cause sagging in the connective tissue known as the *Cooper's ligaments*. So, a good sports bra, whatever your size, is a must. It should feel snug, but not so tight you can't breathe! Seamless or flat seam designs are the best to prevent rubbing.

Just before you head out the door...

"Everyone who has run knows that its most important value is in removing tension and allowing a release from whatever other cares the day may bring."

~Jimmy Carter

You've got your shoes on (and your sports bra, ladies) and you are ready to dive out the door for your first run. Before you do there are some important elements to think about.

If you have had any previous illness or injuries, haven't done any exercise for over a year, suffer with asthma or any other known conditions then it would be best to speak with your doctor before taking up any exercise.

A lot of people decide they want to take up running, go out the door, sprint to the top of the road, collapse in a heap, get back home and think 'not doing that again' and never run again. Not surprising really, and the trick with running is that slow and steady progress is the key to staying injury free and enjoying your running.

First you need to plan – the two main ingredients for any running routine is time and space. The most common reasons I hear for not running are 'I don't have the time' or 'I don't have anywhere to do it'.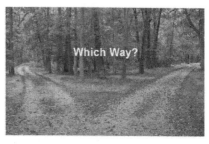
Do you have 30 minutes, 3 times a week? That's all you need. Wherever you can walk you can run. Off road routes (parks, bike paths, playing fields) are better than busy streets and soft surfaces

5

(grass and dirt) are better than paved ones. Map out the best routes in your area and you will save time and make it much more likely you will go out and do your run.

Enlist a friend to come with you, not only does it get you both out the door, it makes the run go quicker when you've got someone else to talk to! (It can also be safer if you're running in pairs)

Kenneth Cooper devised a simple formula to improve as a runner, F.I.T. Frequency (every other day), Intensity (comfortable pace), Time (30 minutes).

When starting out you need to make sure you are running at a comfortable pace, whether you are running for 30 seconds or 30 minutes. What does this mean? A lot of beginners push too hard when they start and get overly tired and discouraged, or even injured. A comfortable pace is when you can talk whilst you are running.

It's OK to walk. Walking during a run is not a form of cheating, it is a common practice among experienced runners during certain types of training to break a big piece of work into smaller sections. Mix running and walking when you're starting to run for the first time, after a long lay-off and to regain fitness after illness or injury.

At the end of this book there is a walk to run 5K training plan that builds slowly week on week and you can monitor your progress as you go through it. This was the type of program I first used when I got back into running.

And then you can progress to the 10K – 12 week training plan! (also at the end of this book!)

Why is the first 10 minutes the hardest...?

"Don't fear moving slowly forward...fear standing still."
~ Kathleen Harris

Whether you're just starting off or have been running a while, one thing you will hear from a group of runners is *'Why is the first 10 minutes the hardest...?* Well here's the science behind what our bodies are doing when we run.

Basically, our body has three energy systems that it uses for the different demands we place on our body.

The *Anaerobic ATP-CP* system – provides us with an immediate boost of energy and it only lasts for 8 – 10 seconds. This energy system does not use oxygen.

The *Anaerobic lactic system* - provides us with another boost of energy which lasts for about 1 – 2 minutes and again does not use oxygen.

The *Aerobic* system - needed for prolonged intensity work. This system provides us with a steady source of energy over a long period of time.

Let us think about how this works when starting to run. Your muscles need a chemical called adenosine triphosphate (ATP) for their energy source. Here's what happens: -

The muscle cells burn off the ATP they have floating around in about 3 seconds.

The next system then kicks in and supplies energy for about 8 – 10 seconds.

If the exercise continues for longer the next system kicks in giving you energy for another 1 – 2 minutes.

Finally, the aerobic system takes over to give you energy over a longer period of time.

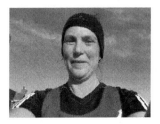

This explains why the first 5 – 10 minutes of exercise can feel quite hard and when you are starting out it is normally in this time that you start to question yourself about what you are doing and if you can do it!

Because your muscles are making demands on your body as you exercise, every system in your body either focuses its efforts on helping the muscles do their work or it shuts down. For example, your heart beats faster during exercise so that it can pump more blood to the muscles, and your stomach shuts down so that it does not waste energy that the muscles can use.

When you run, you will notice that you breathe heavier and faster, your heart beats faster, your muscles hurt and you sweat. This is a normal response to exercise at all levels. When you watch, world-class athletes compete, you see the same responses.

Therefore, the warm up before starting your main exercise is very important – it allows the body and the muscles to get the energy they need to continue.

Now you know what is happening is normal it can make a real difference to how you feel in those first few minutes and continue rather than stop.

The basics of running technique

"If you under-train, you may not finish, but if you over-train, you may not start."

~ Tom DuBos

We all have slightly different running techniques which are individual to us! When you are starting out you do not need to worry about all the different ways – you can explore those later. There are however area's to be aware of which will make sure you are running effectively and with less stress on your body.

Heads up!
Looking forward will mean that you can see where you are going (obvious I know) and it also means your energy is moving forward. If you look down at your feet you are likely to end up on the floor!

Shoulders
You want to relax your shoulders and they should be facing forward, if you start to hunch this will cause tension in the muscles.

Arms
Your arms should be relaxed and have a 90 degree angle at the elbow and your hands at your waist. Many people start off either holding their arms too high or swinging them across their body. This causes tension and uses more energy. If you do find yourself swinging your arms across your body, try thinking about your elbows going back in a straight line behind you.

Hands
Keep your hands relaxed, you can pretend you are lightly holding an egg and don't want to break it.

Overall posture and core muscles

Keep your posture straight. Your shoulders hips and ankles should be aligned (imagine you have a pole through you linking these three areas).

By keeping aligned through the ankle, hips and shoulders you can go faster by leaning forward through the ankles and slow down by leaning back from the ankles – as long as you keep straight.

Feet

You want to be landing on the mid foot and rolling forward onto your toes – landing on your toes can cause pain in the calves and landing on your heel means you are braking on each stride. Try to run with your feet beneath you rather than in front of you.

Breathing

Remember to breathe! This may sound obvious and when we first start running there are some tips to help you get that all important air in as you build up your running you will find what works best for you at different paces.

Breathe in and out through your mouth – you will be able to get more air in.

Breathe from your belly or diaphragm and take short or shallow breathes.

Find out what your normal breathing pattern is by counting your steps. Some runners may find they breathe in for two steps and out for two steps while others may take three steps before the next breath (make sure you are not holding your breath for those steps). Whatever your pattern is, keep it regular and use your steps to monitor your breathing rate.

Listen to your breathing. If you can hear yourself breathing heavily while running at an easy or moderate pace, you are running too quickly for your condition.

Practice slowing down your breathing while running a slower pace before challenging yourself with faster strides.

This may seem like a long list to get started and you can think it through as you run by starting at the top and working down.
So…

Head Up
Shoulders down
Arms and hands relaxed and moving forward
Posture/Body straight
Feet landing under me
Stay relaxed and breathe!

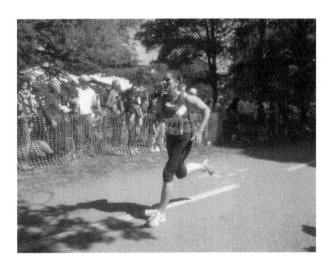

When we get tired it is easy to slump at the shoulders and start bending at the waist. Go through the checklist above to make sure this isn't happening and when you feel yourself slouching, lift your head up and keep your hips forward to keep the alignment through ankles, hips and shoulders. When we start to slump, it means the heart has to work harder to pump the oxygen around to the muscles, also you can find breathing harder as you cannot get all the air you need into the lungs.

You can run faster by increasing your stride turnover, not by overreaching with each stride. On uphill's, shorten your stride and drive more with your arms – you want to maintain an even effort, not pace. When running downhill, again shorten your stride and keep your arms ahead of you for balance and let gravity do the work! With uphill's and downhills, it is important to remember your posture.

As you progress with your running you can look at alternative running techniques with POSE, Chi and Barefoot being the most common alternatives.

To further help and develop your running form there is a chapter on 'Drills for good technique (and form!)'

Warming up for your run

"Begin at the beginning and go on till you come to the end, then stop."

~ Lewis Carroll from Alice in Wonderland

Warming up your muscles before a run or training session is important to prevent injuries. A good warm up means that you will raise your heart rate and start to sweat slightly. This is then followed by some dynamic moves (not stretching as that can cause injuries to the muscles if they are cold.)

Start by walking for 5 minutes, upping the pace to a brisk walk, using your arms as well, once you feel warm you can start doing some 'dynamic movements'. These will help you target the muscles you are about to use.

High Knees
While walking forward at normal pace raise each knee so that it is in line with your hips. Do 10 on each side, turn around and do 10 back.

Heel flicks 1
While moving forward flick your heel up to the underneath of your bottom, keeping your knee at a similar height to your heel and your upper thigh closer to 90 degrees with the floor – this mimics more closely the movement during your run
Do 10 on each side, turn around and do 10 back.

Heel flicks 2
While moving forward 'flick' your heel up to your bottom, keeping your upper thigh straight down in line with your body. Do 10 on each side, turn around and do 10 back.

Grapevine

Moving sideways, start with your feet hip distance apart. Step out to your right side on your right foot. The left leg steps behind the right foot and place the left foot on the ground. Step out to the right again with the right foot and bring the left foot across the front of the right foot and place it on the ground. Repeat 5 times and then lead with the left foot back the other way.

Run backwards

Making sure you have checked the area behind you run backwards (keeping good posture and facing forwards) for 15 steps, turn around and run backwards to the start point.

These movements will make sure your muscles are now ready for your run.

Cool down and stretch

"Take care of your body it's the only place you have to live"
~ Jim Rohn

After your run you need to cool down, bring your heart rate and breathing back to normal level and then stretch out the muscles.

When you have finished your run, move to a brisk walk and over a period of five minutes slow down to normally walking pace. Now is the best time for stretching.

Stretching
There are a couple of rules around stretching for you to get the most from them and prevent injuries.

Never force a stretch or continue it if it causes pain. While pain is to be avoided, to be effective the stretch will cause a sensation of mild discomfort. Be aware while you are stretching of the difference between pain and discomfort.

Hold each stretch for 20 – 30 seconds, while breathing smoothly and concentrating on letting the muscles relax.

Never bounce in a stretch, if you feel you need to deepen the stretch, breathe in and on the out breath gently extend the stretch and hold it in the new position.

Lower Body Stretches
Quadriceps (Quads)

The quadriceps are the muscle in the front of the thigh, and is important for lifting your knees and increasing your speed. Hold a stationary object for balance with one hand and use the opposite hand to grasp the leg on the same side around the ankle, lifting it toward your buttocks. Keep your back straight and your knees together and push forward slightly with your pelvis until you feel the stretch. Change legs.

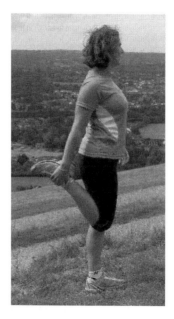

Figure 1 - Quad Stretch

Hamstring stretch

Lie on your back, keeping the back flat and your eyes focused upward. Grasp the back of one thigh with both your hands and (leg bent) pull that thigh into a 90-degree position vs. the floor. Then slowly straighten your knee. After you've gotten used to doing this exercise, you can achieve a better stretch by pulling your thigh closer to your chest—but don't overdo it! Change legs.

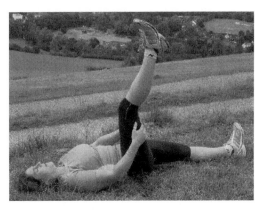

Figure 2 – Hamstring Stretch

Calf stretch

There are two muscles we need to stretch in the calf.

Top of the calf

Stand with your feet hip width apart, move your left foot half a step backwards, slightly bend the left leg and keep the right leg straight. Now bend at the waist keeping your back straight and your head looking forward with your hands resting on the left thigh. You can then raise your bottom and feel the stretch in the top of the calf. Change legs.

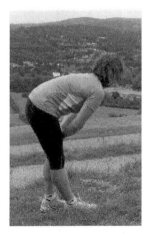

Figure 3 – Top of Calf Stretch

Bottom of the calf

Stand with your feet hip width apart, move your left foot half a step backwards, slightly bend the left leg and keep the right leg straight. Now bend at the waist keeping your back straight and your head looking forward with your hands resting on the left thigh. Raise your toes off the ground and then raise your bottom and feel the stretch in the bottom of the calf. Change legs.

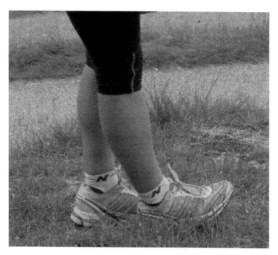

Figure 4 Bottom of Calf Stretch

Upper body stretches

It is just as important to stretch out and release tension from the arms, back and shoulders after a run. Keeping a strong upper body and core is a must for good running technique, especially when you start to feel tired!

Shoulder Stretch

Lift your shoulders up to your ears until you feel the tension in your neck and shoulders. Hold for a count of 10 and then relax your shoulders back down. Repeat 5 times.

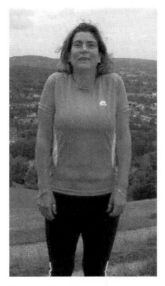

Figure 5 – Shoulder stretch

Upper Back

Stand with feet hip width apart and knees slightly bent. Reach forward with both arms and link hands at chest height. Push arms forward as though 'hugging a tree' to feel the stretch in the upper back.

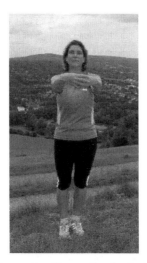

Figure 6 – Upper Back stretch

Upper arm / Triceps

Stand with feet hip width apart, knees slightly bent. Place one hand flat between shoulder blades, keeping the upper arm close to the ear. Using the other arm apply gentle pressure onto the elbow to push hand down back thus assisting with the stretch.

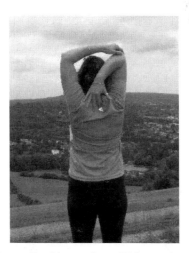

Figure 7 – Upper Arm / Tricep stretch

Getting your mind in your run

"There are people who have no bodies, only heads. And many athletes have no heads, only bodies. A champion is a man who has trained his body and his mind"

~ Coach Sam Dee The Olympian

However much your body might want to go for a run, if your mind isn't interested it's unlikely that you will get out the door.

We can be very good at talking ourselves out of doing something and so when you first start running it's good to think of some outcomes that you want to achieve.

You can break these down from your long term outcome and then smaller ones to keep you on track.

For instance, a long term outcome maybe to take part in a race, do a particular time, fit into a particular pair of jeans.

Your short term outcomes can then be to run 3 times a week, to do a certain amount of mileage in a week, or spend a certain amount of time running each week.

Our brains work really well when it knows what we want to achieve and so if you have a good outcome in place this can help on those days it seems trickier to get out the door!

To create a great outcome think about what you want to achieve and then build up a movie of it in your mind, what can you see happening when you have this outcome, what can you hear and how do you feel. The more detail you can put into this visualisation the more compelling it becomes and the more likely you are to achieve it.

22

By building this vision at the beginning it can mean that on those odd days when you can't be bothered you can bring this vision to the fore and it will help you get out the door.

I have a philosophy that on any given day running can be 10% physical and 90% mental. If you are going to spend time training your body to do what you want it to do, surely the same thinking goes for training your brain!

And that's not just for running....

Staying safe when running

"Runners just do it – they run for the finish line even if someone else has reached it first."

~ Author Unknown

The biggest threat you'll face as a runner on the road, by far, is the car. Traffic zips past you. The best way to lower this risk is to avoid running on roads! For many of us this is just not possible, or it can add time and complexity to our routine. Learn to be extremely cautious on the roads. Try to find quiet roads with wide pavements; run on the right side of the road, facing traffic (the only time to run on the left is if you are on roads without pavements and are coming up to a blind corner i.e. you cannot see round it – so cars will not be able to see you. Make sure you cross back onto the right side of the road as soon as you can safely), obey traffic signs and signals.

I am a big advocate of not running with headphones in but if you are going to then please only have one in so you can still hear what is going on around you.

Make sure you carry some form of identification with you – I have a runner's ID wristband from *RoadID* and if you're a parkrunner you can get one which also has your bar code on it as well! Unfortunately, accidents do happen and if you are involved in one giving the police and paramedics the ability to quickly get in touch with family or friends is vital.

A phone is also a useful item to have with you and most phones these days can fit in the pocket of your shorts or waist bag.

If you are running off road be aware of the terrain, dogs and farm animals – it's always better to go the longer way round a field rather than through a group of animals. They don't know you are out for a run and someone running at them in bright lycra could look a little scary! Always keep your fingers closed in a lightly held fist as fingers out look like a predator's claws and can invoke a reaction.

If you are running at night you must have a Hi-Viz vest which can be bought for about £6 from any running shop. It is also useful to have a head torch which will help you see the paths better and make you more visible to others. This also means you can enjoy running off road on those darker nights

Whether you are running on your own or with someone else it is always worthwhile letting someone know the route you are taking and how long you expect to be, just in case.

It may now seem a little scary to go out with all these things to think about and that is not my intention. I have been out for long runs across the countryside both during the day and at night on my own, as well as running around my local towns and villages and have never had an incident.

By taking a few precautions means that you can enjoy your running without worrying about what's around the next corner!

Running jargon explained

The five S's of sports training are: Stamina, Speed, Strength, Skill and Spirit; but the greatest of these is Spirit.

~ Ken Doherty

As with any sport there are various terms you will hear people talking about that seem to make no sense.

I have listed below the most common terms you will come across in running. This list is not exhaustive!

Carb Loading – Eating extra carbohydrates in the days leading up to a race to give you extra energy.

Fartlek – A Swedish word meaning 'Speed Play'. This term is given to training where you mix up your speed with bursts of fast, medium and slow pace.

Fast/Slow twitch muscles – Two types of muscle fibre. Sprinters are normally made up of more fast twitch muscles and endurance runners have more slow twitch muscles.

Intervals – A type of speed training where you run at race pace or faster for a particular distance and then run/walk slowly for a particular distance and repeat several times.

Lactic Threshold (LT) – The maximum steady state effort that can be maintained without lactate continually increasing.

LSR/LSD – Long slow run/Long slow distance – Running at a comfortable pace where you can have a conversation for a longer distance. Used to build stamina

Perceived effort – From the runner's viewpoint the amount of effort needed to complete a run. A fast run in cool conditions could feel like the same effort of a slow run in hot conditions.

PB – Personal Best – the best time over a set distance.

RICE – The acronym which is used to describe the best way to first treat an injury - Rest, Ice, Compression, Elevate.

Taper – Cutting back on mileage and training in the last few weeks before a big race, to give the muscles rest, usually about 3 weeks before a marathon and 1-2 weeks for a half marathon.

Tempo Run – A form of speed training where you run at an intense pace. These sessions should be hard and not done for a long distance.

Why should I join a running club?

"Stadiums are for spectators. We runners have nature and that is much better."

~ Juha Vaatainen

One of the most common things I hear when speaking to people about running is that they want to wait until they 'are good enough' before joining a running club.

Most running clubs cater for people at all levels of the running spectrum from those just starting up to those running at county level and above.

A club is a great place to meet people who have similar goals and aspirations. You can get support from your fellow runners and give support back.

Knowing that you are going to meet up with other people for your run can also help get you out of the door on days when you are not feeling the love for running!

A lot of clubs also offer training sessions with qualified coaches. Training sessions are much easier to do when you are with other people and someone else is there to help you through the session.

There is also a great social side to many clubs and is a great way to meet other people in your area.

There is a vast amount of knowledge within a running club – from the best races for beginners, training plans devised just for you with a coach, to the best place for a sports massage.

Most clubs will welcome you along for a trial period before you need to commit to join and a lot of them are far cheaper than gyms and you can also get reduced race entry fees and discounts at local running shops.

If you live in an area that doesn't have a local running club there is a great on-line community that you can get support from. The best I have found is *Fetcheveryone.com* which is a club you can join to get the benefits listed above and has loads of information and support on line. There are forums for discussions and areas to record your training and see your improvements.

Although I belong to a running club, I use the website and enjoy the forums.

parkruns – although not a club, these are free 5K measured and timed runs that take place every Saturday morning up and down the country. They are a great place to meet other runners and were set up for people of all abilities. All you need to do is go online and register, you get emailed back a barcode which you take along when you run. They are a great way to measure your progress as you train and improve.

So, what are you waiting for? Look up your local club and get down there today!

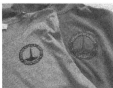

What should I be eating?

"I run so my goals in life will continue to get bigger instead of my belly."

~ Bill Kirby

Sports nutrition is a big topic. However, in general the rules for good nutrition and fluid intake are the same for runners as everyone else. There are three areas that are of particular interest to runners.

1. Controlling weight – extra pounds will add time to your run and put your body under added stress.
2. Eat something small in the 20 minutes after training or racing – a protein bar or banana for example.
3. Drink 250 – 500ml of water or energy drink in the hour or so before running to help prevent dehydration.

Eating healthily will help your body refuel and have the energy to do your training. Be careful of falling into the trap of 'I've done a run, so now I can eat this very large piece of gooey chocolate cake, I deserve it!' Doing that after every run is not going to help you lose or maintain your weight. A treat once a week for rewarding yourself for the work that you have done is great, just not every day!

As a runner, you need to make sure you are getting a good balance of the following: -

Carbohydrates - Whole grain pasta, steamed or boiled rice, potatoes, fruits, starchy vegetables, and whole grain breads are all good carb sources

Protein - lean meats, fish, low-fat dairy products, poultry, whole grains, and beans.

Fat - nuts, oils, and cold-water fish provide essential fats called omega-3s.

Calcium - low-fat dairy products, calcium-fortified juices, dark leafy vegetables, beans, and eggs.

Eating well will give you all the energy you need to train at your optimum level.

For Ultra runners being able to eat and run is very important and so you need to test out different foods on your runs (any excuse...)

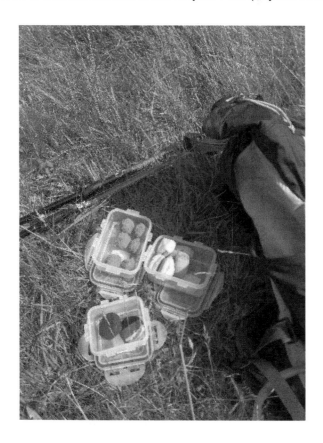

Popular road and trail distances

"It's very hard in the beginning to understand that the whole idea is not to beat the other runners. Eventually you learn that the competition is against the little voice inside you that wants you to quit."

~ George Sheehan

Distances

There is a wide variety of race distances out in the world and the following are the most common.

5 kilometres
5 miles
10 kilometres
10 miles
Half marathon (13.1 miles)
Marathon (26.2 miles)
Ultra – (anything over 26.2 miles)

People often start off with a 5K race, the **Race for Life** and **parkruns** are both this distance.

As you conquer each distance you then tend to move up to the next one and it can be very rewarding to look back when you have done a 10K and remember how you found your first 5K and how much you have improved.

There are those who go straight into a Marathon, London being one of the most well known for raising money for Charity. There are however many, many other marathons around the country which can offer the challenge of training and a better chance of running for a time.

Types
Road Running
Any run or race that takes place on road or pavement! The distances for races range from 5 kilometres up to Marathon.

Cross Country/Trail/Fell
Any run or race that is off road and on natural terrain with distances from 5K to Ultra, these happen all year round. Cross Country races are traditionally run in the Autumn and Winter. Running off road can be more testing to a runner as the terrain can change from trail, to woodland, to grass, to ploughed field all in a matter of minutes. It is however to my mind much more rewarding than road running

Track running
Any run or race on a running track, this can be grass or synthetic. The distances range from the sprints of 100 meters up to middle distance of 1500 metres. You will also see at championships that the 5 kilometres and 10 kilometre races are also done on the track.

Whatever distance or type you pick remember the hard work is in the training – getting out the door to do your runs on a regular basis is the key that can unlock your potential!

Whatever surface you normally train on if you have booked a race you want to be aiming for at least 50% of your training on the type of surface the race will be on. This gives your mind and body a chance to adjust and get used to it. For instance, if you book a road race but always train on the trails the hard tarmac surface could cause you problems and injuries in the race.

Common injuries

*"If you run 100 miles a week, you can eat anything you want –
Why? Because… (a) You'll burn all the calories you consume, (b)
you deserve it and (c) you'll be injured soon and back on a
restricted diet anyway."*

~ Don Kardong

As with any sport, injuries can occur when running. Most injuries
are musculoskeletal which means we can recover quickly if we take
time off and take appropriate action – e.g. RICE (Rest, Ice,
Compression, Elevate). They can also be self inflicted, running too
far, too fast, too soon or too often!

You can help yourself by:-
Wearing the right shoes
Building up your training slowly
Warm up and stretch afterwards
Keeping good posture when running
Varying your running surface
Eat well and stay hydrated
Get regular sports massage
Listen to what your body is telling you.

Some of the most common injuries are: -
Shin Splints – this term covers a broad range of pain that is felt
along the front lower leg. Wearing the right footwear can help
prevent this. A physiotherapist can help you find the exact cause.

Achilles Tendonitis – This tendon runs from the large calf muscle
to your heel and helps you push off when you run. To help prevent
this vary your running surface and include calf stretches into your
routine.

Iliotibial band syndrome (ITBS) also known as Runners Knee - The Iliotibial band is a sheath of thick, fibrous connective tissue which attaches at the top to the hip bone and Tensor fascia latae muscle. It then runs down the outside of the thigh and inserts into the outer surface of the Tibia (shin bone). Its purpose is to extend the knee joint (straighten it) as well as to abduct the hip (move it out sideways).

As the ITB passes over the bony part on the outside of the knee (lateral epicondyle) it can be prone to friction. At an angle of approximately 20-30 degrees the IT band flicks across the lateral epicondyle. When the knee is being straightened it flicks in front of the epicondyle and when it is bent, it flicks back behind. This is a problem for runners as 20 – 30 degrees is the approximate angle the knee is at when the foot strikes the ground when running! To help prevent this regularly stretch the hip flexors and massage along the IT Band.

Knee pain can be caused by a variety of reasons but one of the most overlooked is an imbalance in the strength of muscles running down the outside and inside of your thigh. This can cause the knee to be pulled more in one direction that the other. Make sure you stretch both the inner and outer muscles after training and if you are using weights machines that you build up both. Knee pain can also be caused by problems in the hips and piriformis muscle so making sure you warm up well and stretch out afterwards can help.

Plantar fasciitis is when you strain the plantar fascia, which is the tissue which supports your foot arch and runs from the heel to your toes. It can become weak swollen or irritated/inflamed. If you have this then rest is the first thing you need to do and treatment with a physio can help the healing process.

Top 5 myths about running

"Tough times don't last but tough people do."

~ A.C. Green

Myth 1 - Runners don't need strength training

Strength training improves your injury resistance, your running strength, your muscle elasticity and your running economy. It makes you a better, faster, more efficient runner. You will not become muscle bound -endurance training won't allow it.

Myth 2 - Static stretching should be done before you run.

Static stretching cold muscles is more likely to result in injury and may reduce your muscles ability during training. Dynamic movements during your warm up is much more effective and then leave the static stretching for after your training.

Myth 3 – Sore muscles are caused by lactic acid build up.

Sore muscles after a run are actually caused by microscopic tears in your muscles. This is why we have rest days as the tears heal and this results in stronger muscles!

Myth 4 – You shouldn't walk during a run

There is nothing wrong with walking during a run. Not every run needs to be at a hard pace. It can aid recovery to make sure you can do the next piece of training and if you're running through the countryside it can be very nice to stop and take in what's around you. It all depends on your outcome for that particular session.

Myth 5 - You aren't a runner until you've completed a marathon

Rubbish – Anyone that gets out the door and runs is a runner. It doesn't matter on the distance or speed.

Walk to run 5K in 12 weeks

Make sure you warm up before each training session and stretch AFTER you have completed the session.

	Monday	Thursday	Saturday
Week 1	Run 2 mins walk 4 mins **Repeat x 3**	Run 2 mins walk 4 mins **Repeat x 3**	Run 2 mins walk 4 mins **Repeat x 3**
Week 2	Run 2 mins Walk 4 mins **Repeat x 5**	Run 2 mins Walk 4 mins **Repeat x 5**	Run 2 mins Walk 4 mins **Repeat x 5**
Week 3	Run 3 mins Walk 3 mins **Repeat x 4**	Run 3 mins Walk 3 mins **Repeat x 4**	Run 3 mins Walk 3 mins **Repeat x 4**
Week 4	Run 5 mins Walk 3 mins **Repeat x 3**	Run 5 mins Walk 3 mins **Repeat x 3**	Run 5 mins Walk 3 mins **Repeat x 3**
Week 5	Run 7 mins Walk 2 mins **Repeat x 3**	Run 7 mins Walk 2 mins **Repeat x 3**	Run 7 mins Walk 2 mins **Repeat x 3**
Week 6	Run 8 mins Walk 2 mins **Repeat x 3**	Run 8 mins Walk 2 mins **Repeat x 3**	Run 8 mins Walk 2 mins **Repeat x 3**
Week 7	Run 8 mins Walk 2 mins **Repeat x 3**	Run 10 mins Walk 2 mins **Repeat x 2**	Run 10 mins Walk 2 mins **Repeat x 2**
Week 8	Run 10 mins Walk 2 mins **Repeat x 2**	Run 10 mins Walk 2 mins **Repeat x 2** Then Run 5 mins	Run 10 mins Walk 2 mins **Repeat x 2** Then Run 5 mins
Week 9	Run 12 mins Walk 2 mins **Repeat x 2**	Run 12 mins Walk 2 mins **Repeat x 2** Then Run 5 mins	Run 12 mins Walk 2mins **Repeat x 2** Then Run 5 mins

	Monday	Thursday	Saturday
Week 10	Run 12 mins Walk 2 mins **Repeat x 2** Then Run 5 mins	Run 15 mins Walk 1 mins **Repeat x 2**	Run 15 mins Walk 1 mins **Repeat x 2**
Week 11	Run 15 mins Walk 1 mins **Repeat x 2**	Run 15 mins Walk 1 mins **Repeat x 2** Then Run 5 mins	Run 15 mins Walk 1 mins **Repeat x 2** Then Run 5 mins
Week 12	Run 15 mins Walk 1 mins **Repeat x 2** Then Run 5 mins	Run 20 mins Walk 1 mins **Repeat x 2**	run until you need a break, aiming to run for 30 mins without stopping.

If you are not racing on the last day of week 12 then continue to train 3 times per week making sure the increase for each week is no more than 10% of time or distance (not both at the same time) from the previous week. The week in the run up to the race you need to taper down and I would repeat day one of week 12 twice that week making sure you have a rest break of at least 2 – 3 days from the last day of training.

Moving up to 10K

Make sure you warm up before each training session and stretch AFTER you have completed the session.

	Tuesday	Thursday	Saturday	Sunday
Week 1	Warm up 8 x 4 mins 2 mins recovery	3 miles easy pace	parkrun or 3 miles fast pace	45 minutes relaxed run
Week 2	Warm up 5 x 6 mins 2 mins recovery	3.5 miles easy pace	parkrun or 3 miles fast pace	50 minutes relaxed run
Week 3	Warm up 9 x 4 mins 2 mins recovery	4 miles easy pace	parkrun or 3 miles fast pace	60 minutes relaxed run
Week 4	Warm up 6 x 6 mins 2 mins recovery	4.5 miles easy pace	parkrun or 3 miles fast pace	55 minutes relaxed run
Week 5	Warm up 10 x 4 mins 2 mins recovery	3.5 miles easy pace	parkrun or 3 miles fast pace	65 minutes relaxed run
Week 6	Warm up 7 x 6 mins 2 mins recovery	4 miles easy pace	parkrun or 3 miles fast pace	70 minutes relaxed run
Week 7	Warm up 11 x 4 mins 2 mins recovery	4.5 miles easy pace	parkrun or 3 miles fast pace	60 minutes relaxed run

	Tuesday	Thursday	Saturday	Sunday
Week 8	Warm up 4 x 8 mins 2 mins recovery	5 miles easy pace	parkrun or 3 miles fast pace	70 minutes relaxed run
Week 9	Warm up 5 x 8 mins 2 mins recovery	4 miles easy pace	parkrun or 3 miles fast pace	80 minutes relaxed run
Week 10	Warm up 4 x 10 mins 2 mins recovery	4.5 miles easy pace	parkrun or 3 miles fast pace	55 minutes relaxed run
Week 11	Warm up 10 x 4 mins 2 mins recovery	5 miles easy pace	parkrun or 3 miles fast pace	45 minutes relaxed run
Week 12	Warm up 8 x 4 mins 2 mins recovery	4 miles easy pace	Rest day	RACE DAY!

Easy pace – A pace you can have a conversation with someone.

Fast pace – You can get a few words out but cannot hold a conversation

Relaxed – this will be close to your easy pace - the focus is on making sure you stay relaxed throughout the run as this is your longest run each week.

Tuesday session – the main part of the session to be done as hard efforts – so either a fast pace or perhaps find a hill to do them on – in which case it's not about your speed it is about your effort! The sessions work as interval session so for the first week you will run hard effort for 4 minutes and then have 2 minutes walking recovery before doing the next 4 minutes, and you repeat 8 times.

If you are not racing on the last day of week 12 then continue to train 4 times per week making sure the increase for each week is no more than 10% of time or distance (not both at the same time) from the previous week.

Drills and techniques for good running form

These drills can be used as some of your dynamic movements during your warm up.

It is also worth using one of your run sessions every few weeks to concentrate just on the drills to help you hone down the techniques and give your mind and body a chance to really feel and understand what it is you are asking of it.

By creating your own great running form will help you run more relaxed, which will make you faster and help prevent injuries.

Do these drills over a distance of about 10 meters. If you are using them as your dynamic movements then do them twice each, if you are doing them as full session then 5 – 10 times making sure you are fully in control of the movement.

Ankles
Shuffling forward with small steps concentrating on working ankles by raising onto tip toes.

- Take tiny steps moving each foot just slightly ahead of the other
- Have very little knee raise
- Think about each foot moving from fully on the floor to up onto the toes.
- Use your arms in time with your feet.
- Play with the speed of the movement

You can vary this drill by raising your knees to waist height so that your foot leaves the floor.

High knees
Small steps, knee's coming up to waist height

- Exaggerate your normal running action so that your knees lift to waist height
- Use your arms in a strong even swing
- Keep your leg movements fast
- Place one foot down just in front of the other
- Maintain a strong core, keeping yourself straight through the shoulders and hips.

Skipping
Skipping with height and skipping with forward momentum

Height
- Using arms skip as high as you can moving forward a short distance.
- Raise knee to at least waist height
- Exaggerate your arm movements
- At the end of the 10 meters move into a few meters of normal running.

Forward
- Using your arms skip as far forward as you can (bounding forward)
- Raise knee to at least waist height
- Exaggerate your arm movements
- At the end of the 10 meters move into a few meters of normal running.

Forward kicks

Starting with a skipping motion and putting your focus into kicking your leg forward through the movement.

- Keep a strong core although you can have a slight lean forward (to stop you leaning backwards!) making sure you do not twist at your hips.
- Use the full foot range of motion.

Heel flicks

Heel flicks 1

- Moving forward flick your heel up to the underneath of your bottom
- Keep your knee at a similar height to your heel and your upper thigh closer to 90 degrees with the floor
- At the end of the 10 meters move into a few meters of normal running.

Heel flicks 2

- Moving forward 'flick' your heel up to your bottom
- Keep your knee pointing down
- Keep your upper thigh straight down in line with your body.
- At the end of the 10 meters move into a few meters of normal running.

Running jumps

Bounding strides, like the middle phase of a triple jump.

- Lengthen your normal running stride by driving the knee forward
- Use your arms to help exaggerate the movement
- At the end of the 10 meters move into a few meters of normal running.

Fast feet

Very quick movement of the feet

- Very short fast steps, lifting off the ground quickly.
- Use your arms to help the feet move quickly
- The foot must leave the ground
- Maintain a strong core, keeping yourself straight through the shoulders and hips.
- At the end of the 10 meters move into a few meters of normal running.

Hops

- Using both legs jump forward for 10 meters and then backwards to your starting point.
- Do the same hopping on your right leg and then switch to your left leg.
- On your right leg hop 10 metres sideways and then back to the start and the switch to your left leg.

Squats

You may want to do these over 5 metres to start with!

- Squat with feet and knees together, step sideways with your right leg and back and then with your left.
- Squat with legs shoulder width apart. Cross your right foot over your left foot, then step your left foot out to the left, repeat
- Squat with legs shoulder width apart. Cross your right foot in front of your left, then step your left foot out and then step your right foot behind your left and step your left foot out again (known as a grapevine) keeping in the squat position.

Core Exercises

You don't need to go to a gym to develop a strong core. Having a strong core will help you keep your running form when you are tired, which helps you run longer, stronger faster and stay injury free.

I love these exercises and you can do them twice a week. In order to mix them up and stop the sessions from becoming boring I suggest you put them in a hat and pick out 8 to do, you can then do the next 8 on your next core day. Putting them all back in and ready to lucky dip the next week.

Start with a light warm up for a few minutes, for example marching on the spot and swinging the arms for 2 minutes. The goal of the warm up is to get your blood circulating and your body temperature rising in order to prepare for higher intensity exercise.

Perform each exercise for 30 seconds to two minutes depending upon your conditioning. Move to the next exercise smoothly, but quickly. You can continue the routine as long as you like (a twenty minute workout or an hour or more). Cool down with five or more minutes of stretching.

1. **Push Ups**

   Begin in push up position, on knees or toes. Perform 4 push ups, abs in and back straight. On the 5th push up, lower halfway down and hold for 4 counts. Push back up and repeat the series - 4 regular push ups and 1 halfway--5 or more times.

2. **One-Leg Balance / Squat / Reach**

   Stand on one leg and hold it as long as you can. If this is too easy, add a slight squat motion. Still too easy? Place an object on the floor, several feet in front of you (a book, perhaps), and slowly squat down, and reach out with one arm and touch the object and slowly return to an upright position. Stay on one leg at all times. Repeat on the other leg after a minute or so.

3. **Wall Sit**

   With your back against a wall, and your feet about 2 feet away from the wall, slide down until your knees are at a 90 degree angle. Hold the position as long as you can. This is great for ski conditioning.

4. **Abdominal Crunches**

   Lie on your back with your knees bent and feet flat on the floor. Place your fingertips to the side of your head just behind your ears. Push your lower back into the floor flattening the arch and hold. Curl up slowly so both your shoulders lift off the floor a few inches. Hold for a count of 2 and return to the start position. Tip: Don't tuck your chin to your chest; keep your head up.

5. **Supermans**

   Lie on your stomach with your arms and legs stretched out. Raise your arms and legs off the ground a few inches, hold a few seconds, and then lower. Alternate arms and legs as an option. Repeat.

6. **Reverse Crunch**

   Lie on your back with your hands out to your sides, and bend your knees. Bring your knees toward your head until your hips come up slightly off the floor (don't rock). Hold one second, put your feet slowly back down and repeat.

7. **Squat-Thrusts**

   Stand with feet together. Squat down and place your hands on the floor next to your feet. In an explosive movement, jump feet backwards into a push-up position, jump feet back between hands and stand up.

8. Jumping Jacks

The basic jumping jack is a good cardio and strength training exercise.

9. Side Jumps

Stand with feet together. Jump to the right several feet, keeping knees bent and landing in a squat position. Jump back to the left and continue jumping from side to side. Use a small object to jump over if you like (book, pillow etc.)

10. Mountain Climbers

Start on your hands and knees and get into in a sprinter's start position. Keep your hands on the ground and push off with your feet so you alternate foot placement (run in place) as long as you can. Be sure to keep your back straight, not arched.

11. Wall Squat-Thrusts

Lean into a wall with your hands and keep your feet shoulder width apart several feet from the wall. Slowly lift one knee up toward your chest and back and then the other leg. As you improve your fitness, increase your leg lift speed and move your weight onto the ball of the rear foot.

12. Backward Stride

Stand with feet together. Stride backward with one leg, while raising the arms to shoulder level. Lower the arms to your side and repeat with the other leg. Pick up the pace for more cardio.

13. Jump Lunges

Start in the lunge position – one foot forward with knee bent over the heel and one foot back with the back knee just above the floor. Bend your knees and then jump up high and switch leg positions. Use explosive, but controlled movements.

14. Walking Lunge

Start in the lunge position at one end of the room and take a long stride forward with the right leg. Bend down so the forward knee is directly over the heel and at a 90 degree angle. Raise up and repeat with the other leg across the room.

15. Pull Ups

The pull up exercise does require some basic equipment, or some creativity (go to a playground or find a low hanging tree branch, for example), but it's a great, simple way to build upper body strength.

With both hands on the bar, pull your body up so that your chin is level with the bar.

If you are just starting you can use a chair so that you start in the up position and lower yourself down slowly (do not let yourself fall using gravity as that's using momentum not muscles!), as you grow stronger you will be able to pull up rather than lower down.

16. Chair Dips

You'll need two chairs, (or a bed and a chair or a counter, etc....) for this great tricep exercise. Place two chairs facing each other, about 3 feet apart. Sit on one chair with your hands palm down and gripping the edge of the chair. Place your heels on the edge of the other chair and hold yourself up using your triceps. Slide forward just far enough that your behind clears the edge of the chair and lower yourself so your elbows are at 90 degrees. Do as many repetitions as you can.

The Quitter

When you're lost on the trail with the speed of a snail
And defeat looks you straight in the eye,
and you're needing to sit, your whole being says quit
You're certain it's your time to die.
But the code of the trail is "move forward don't fail"
Though your knees and ego are scarred.
All the swelling and pain is just part of the game
In the long run it's quitting that's hard!
"I'm sick of the pain!"
Well, now, that's a shame
But you're strong, you're healthy, and bright.
So you've had a bad stretch and you're ready to retch,
Shoulders back, move forward, and fight.
It's the plugging away that will win you the day,
Now don't be a loser my friend!
So the goal isn't near, why advance to the rear.
All struggles eventually end.
It's simple to cry that you're finished; and die.
It's easy to whimper and whine.
Move forward and fight, though there's no help in sight you'll soon
cross the lost finish line.
You'll come out of the black, with the wind at your back,
As the clouds start to part; there's the sun.
Then you'll know in your heart, as you did at the start.
You're not a quitter.
You've Won!!

Gene Thibeault

About the Author

"You have to wonder at times what you're doing out there. Over the years, I've given myself a thousand reason to keep running, but it always comes back to where it started. It comes down to self-satisfaction and a sense of achievement."

~ *Steve Prefontaine*

Annie Page is The ULTRA Coach giving you the EDGE in Business, Sport, Life

Bringing together the most effective disciplines from both Business and Sport so that everyone can benefit by learning and applying them to deliver success.

I work with people who want to achieve their best and who want to excel in their environment.

Using Focus, Motivation and Analysis to bring you success for your business, your sport, your life.

With Annie Page – The ULTRA Coach giving you the EDGE you will go beyond your limitations and develop your full potential.

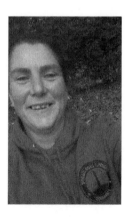

Sport

I work with competitors, coaches, clubs and National Governing Bodies across a range of sporting disciplines using coaching and training techniques to focus on getting results and to achieve peak performance.

By understanding mental strategies and thinking patterns that are used to be able to make decisions in the moment that will enhance performance.

As a UK Athletics Endurance running coach I create individual and bespoke training plans with ongoing support so that you will reach your goals from 5K to Ultra's!

Business Blueprint

Using a 12-week programme to deliver success your business will benefit by breaking down long term goals into 12 week phased wins. Each phase has specific aims to create development and achieve success.

In the same way athletes split their long-term goals into more manageable phases of training giving time to Focus, Motivate and Analyse so your long-term business goals will become a series of achievements.

Life

Helping people utilise the skills they have and develop and fine tune them as their own techniques and resources to support them to achieve their goals. Individuals learn more about themselves and how they can take the skills and techniques into other areas of their life.

www.anniepage.co.uk

How I got started...

"Having not run since leaving school, where I was probably one of the few who actually enjoyed cross country. I started running again in 2004, with a friend and we started off not being able to run for more than a couple of minutes and then needing to walk, which was great because the plan we were following told us to do just that (there is one in this book and you've just gone past it).

From there I fell back in love with running, with racing and getting out in the fresh air and enjoying the countryside. I joined my local club **Ampthill and Flitwick Flyers** and enjoy the camaraderie that belonging to a club gives.

I wanted to give something back to the club and so became a coach and have attended various UK Athletics run courses over the last few years to keep my knowledge up to date.

As well as regularly coaching with the Nice & Easies group at the club, I am also proud to have been part of the 'Get back into running' team with **TeamBEDS&LUTON** in 2008, where I devised and delivered the program. This won an England Athletics partnership award for **Ampthill & Flitwick Flyers** and **TeamBeds&Luton**.

With my company I have enjoyed using my coaching and training skills to work with Leaders in companies, run management training courses and work with individuals to achieve their outcomes and goals. I also coach sports teams and individuals working with them as they focus on getting results and training their brain so that mind and body are working together to achieve peak performance.

I continue with my own personal development to bring new thinking and develop new skills to share with those I work with.

Running has helped me find a balance in which to let my competitive side thrive. I run against myself, what I think my limitations are, and push the boundaries further back each time.

I have now found a great love of off road Ultra's and enjoy the self navigation and challenge that these bring. My longest run so far has been a 100 miler from Wadebridge, Cornwall to Teignmouth, Devon and I am planning on continuing with both 'all in one go' Ultra's and multi day events.

Good luck and enjoy your running.

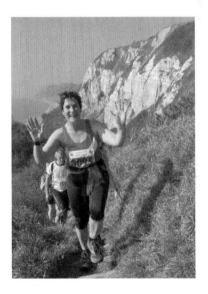

Update

Having moved down to Cornwall in 2015 I have also changed running clubs and now run with Bodmin Road Runners, another very friendly, enthusiastic and fun running club and I enjoy being part of the club and coaching.

The main difference now is that my trails have got a lot hillier and I'm never far from the coastal path and the most amazing scenery!

Thank you's

Andrew Gatland from *SuspendDisbelief* for the photographs of me in the stretching section– even though he did make me run up Box Hill more than a few times! Get in touch with him at: *www.suspenddisbelief.co.uk*

My great friends in the Nice and Easies and Ampthill and Flitwick Flyers Running Club for various quotes and pieces of advice during the last few years and those specifically to add to this book. And for being such great company to run with!

Bodmin Road Runners, for their fab welcome and helping to keep my enthusiasm and love of all things running.

Martin Bennett and Lucy Hampton for their initial feedback on the book.

Jane Miles for first agreeing to start running with me in 2004.

Carl French at The Endless Bookcase for encouraging me to write this book and supporting me with advice and humour.

Postface

(Not a preface 'cos it's at the back!)

The picture below shows where the leg muscles mentioned in this book are.

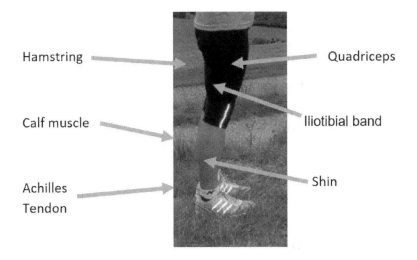

Hamstring

Quadriceps

Calf muscle

Iliotibial band

Achilles Tendon

Shin

Jargon, science and technical terms

Aerobic – energy system meaning 'with oxygen' – it has become the word to use for any physical exercise

Anaerobic – energy system meaning 'not using oxygen'

ATP – a molecule called adenosine triphosphate which produces energy

CP – a molecule called creatine phosphate which helps restore ATP

Lactic system – releases energy to ATP

Endorphins – endogenous morphine – small protein molecules produced during exercise, when feeling fear, being in love – known as giving a feeling of well being

NLP – Neuro Linguistic Programming

Coopers Ligament – connective tissue in the breast which helps maintain structural integrity.

Printed in Great Britain
by Amazon